The Bethesda System

Springer
New York
Berlin
Heidelberg
Barcelona
Budapest
Hong Kong
London
Milan
Paris
Santa Clara
Singapore
Tokyo

Robert J. Kurman
Diane Solomon

The Bethesda System for Reporting Cervical/Vaginal Cytologic Diagnoses

Definitions, Criteria, and Explanatory Notes for Terminology and Specimen Adequacy

With 61 color illustrations

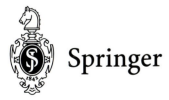

Springer

Robert J. Kurman
Johns Hopkins University
School of Medicine
Baltimore, MD 21287
USA

Diane Solomon
National Cancer Institute
Bethesda, MD 20892
USA

Library of Congress Cataloging-in-Publication Data
The Bethesda system for reporting cervical/vaginal cytologic diagnoses
  : definitions, criteria and explanatory notes for terminology and
  specimen adequacy / Robert Kurman, Diane Solomon.
        p.   cm.
    ISBN 0-387-94077-4. — ISBN 3-540-94077-4 (Berlin)
    1. Cervix uteri—Cytopathology—Terminology.   2. Vagina—
—Cytopathology—Terminology.   3. Cervix uteri—Diseases—
—Cytodiagnosis—Terminology.   4. Vagina—Diseases—Cytodiagnosis—
—Terminology.   I. Kurman, Robert J.
    [DNLM: 1. Cervix Diseases—diagnosis.   2. Cervix Diseases—
—classification.   3. Vaginal Diseases—diagnosis.   4. Vaginal
Diseases—classification.   5. Cytodiagnosis—methods.
6. Cytological Techniques.   WP 470 B562 1993]
RG310. B48 1993
618. 1′ 407—dc20
DNLM/DLC   93-31572

Printed on acid-free paper.

Production managed by Jim Harbison; manufacturing supervised by Rhea Talbert.
Typeset by ATLIS Graphics and Design, Inc., Mechanicsburg, PA.
Printed and bound by Walsworth Publishing Co., Marceline, MO.
Printed in the United States of America.

9 8 7 6 5

ISBN 0-387-94077-4 Springer-Verlag New York Berlin Heidelberg
ISBN 3-540-94077-4 Springer-Verlag Berlin Heidelberg New York

Contents

Contributors

Robert J. Kurman, M.D.*†
Chairman, Criteria Committee
Johns Hopkins University, Baltimore, MD

Ronald D. Luff, M.D., M.P.H.*
Chairman, Editorial Committee
Sacred Heart Hospital, Allentown, PA

Barbara F. Atkinson, M.D.†
Medical College of Pennsylvania, Philadelphia, PA

Jonathan S. Berek, M.D.*
University of California at Los Angeles School of Medicine,
Los Angeles, CA

Marluce Bibbo, M.D., Sc.D.*
Thomas Jefferson University, Philadelphia, PA

Thomas A. Bonfiglio, M.D.†
University of Rochester, Rochester, NY

Christopher P. Crum, M.D.†
Brigham and Women's Hospital, Boston, MA

Yener S. Erozan, M.D.†
Johns Hopkins University, Baltimore, MD

Yao Shi Fu, M.D.†
University of California at Los Angeles, Los Angeles, CA

Shirley E. Greening, M.S., J.D.*
Thomas Jefferson University, Philadelphia, PA

Michael R. Henry, M.D.†
National Naval Medical Center, Bethesda, MD

Donald E. Henson, M.D.*
National Cancer Institute, Bethesda, MD

Mujtaba Husain, M.D.†
Sinai Hospital, Detroit, MI

Robert V. P. Hutter, M.D.*
St. Barnabas Medical Center, Livingston, NJ

Stanley L. Inhorn, M.D.*
University of Wisconsin, Madison, WI

Howard W. Jones III, M.D.*
Vanderbilt University Medical Center, Nashville, TN

Nancy B. Kiviat, M.D.†
University of Washington, Seattle, WA

Tilde S. Kline, M.D.†
Lankenau Hospital, Wynnewood, PA

Paul A. Krieger, M.D.*
MetPath Inc., Teterboro, NJ

George D. Malkasian, Jr., M.D.*
Mayo Clinic, Rochester, MN

Alexander Meisels, M.D.†
Hôpital du Saint-Sacrement, Quebec City, PQ

Mary L. Nielsen, M.D.*
Pathology Consultants, Wichita, KS

Stanley F. Patten, Jr., M.D., Ph.D.
University of Rochester, Rochester, NY

Vincent P. Perna, M.D.*
SmithKline Beecham Laboratories, St. Louis, MO

Dorothy L. Rosenthal, M.D.*
University of California at Los Angeles School of Medicine,
Los Angeles, CA

Patricia E. Saigo, M.D.*
Memorial Sloan-Kettering Cancer Center, New York, NY

Alexander Sedlis, M.D.*
State University of New York Health Science Center at Brooklyn,
Brooklyn, NY

Mark E. Sherman, M.D.
Johns Hopkins University, Baltimore, MD

Diane Solomon, M.D.*†
National Cancer Institute, Bethesda, MD

Theresa Somrak, C.T.(ASCP), J.D.
Cytopathology Education Consortium, Chicago, IL

Leo B. Twiggs, M.D.*
University of Minnesota, Minneapolis, MN

George L. Wied, M.D.*
University of Chicago, Chicago, IL

---

*Denotes members of The Bethesda System Editorial Committee
†Denotes members of The Bethesda System Criteria Committee

Introduction

The Bethesda System (TBS) for Reporting Cervical/Vaginal Cytologic Diagnoses was developed at a National Cancer Institute (NCI)–sponsored workshop in December 1988 to provide uniform diagnostic terminology that would facilitate communication between the laboratory and the clinician. The format of TBS report includes a descriptive diagnosis and an evaluation of specimen adequacy. TBS was designed to be flexible so that it could evolve in response to changing needs in cervical cancer screening as well as to advances in the field of cervical pathology. Subsequently, a second workshop was held in April 1991 to evaluate the impact of TBS in actual practice and to amend and modify it where needed. One of the major recommendations of this second meeting was that precise criteria should be formulated for both the diagnostic terms and for the descriptors of specimen adequacy. That is the intended purpose of this monograph.

The classification used in TBS is not a histogenetic one, but rather a nomenclature designed to facilitate categorization and reporting of cytologic diagnoses. The overall diagnosis, as in the World Health Organization (WHO) system, is based on the most abnormal cells present regardless of their number. In addition, it should be noted that the site of origin of an abnormality detected in a cervical/vaginal cytologic sample cannot always be specified because morphologically identical tumors may arise in the vagina, cervix, endometrium, or ovary.

The criteria and descriptions provided in this monograph are intended to supplement the classification and are not meant to be a comprehensive treatise on gynecologic cytopathology. For a detailed discussion the reader is directed to several comprehensive cytopathology textbooks. Use of these criteria should facilitate uniform application of TBS and result in more consistent reporting of cytologic diagnoses. However, it should be emphasized that cervical/vaginal cytopathology includes an element of subjective interpretation and consequently the application of these criteria should be viewed within this context.

The Bethesda System

Part 1

Specimen Adequacy

Definitions, Criteria, and Explanatory Notes

Background

The incorporation of specimen adequacy as an integral part of the report has been widely acknowledged as one of the most important contributions of TBS. The 1988 Bethesda System listed potential reasons for designating a specimen other than fully *Satisfactory* but did not incorporate specific criteria for the evaluation of specimen adequacy. Participants at the 1991 Bethesda System Workshop and others in the cytopathology community voiced the need for guidance in this area. In response, the Criteria Committee was charged with the development of morphologic criteria for the evaluation of adequacy.

The following guidelines represent the consensus of several experts in the field of cytopathology based on a combination of experience and review of a relatively sparse scientific database. The criteria, therefore, should be viewed as an initial attempt to develop a more standardized approach to the evaluation of adequacy. Dissemination of these criteria, it is hoped, may serve as an impetus for additional studies to address remaining critical questions regarding valid measures of specimen adequacy. Modification of these guidelines may be required as a result of these studies.

Four elements constitute the adequacy of the specimen for the detection of abnormalities of the uterine cervix: (1) patient and specimen identification, (2) pertinent clinical information, (3) technical interpretability, and, (4) cellular composition and sampling of the transformation zone.

Patient and Specimen Identification

Besides the obvious need for correct specimen identification, proper identification of the patient allows the laboratory to locate prior records and slides that may influence the current evaluation.

Pertinent Clinical Information

Provision of pertinent clinical information to the cytopathologist can improve the reliability of the evaluation. These data may clarify otherwise uncertain cytologic findings, and laboratories often use this information to select cases for special review. Since a specimen lacking pertinent clinical information may not receive the extent of review or clinical correlation it would have received had that information been provided, TBS places it in the "Satisfactory but limited" category.

Technical Interpretability

The cellular constituents must be interpretable for diagnostic evaluation. A variety of factors may impair or prevent such interpretation (see criteria below).

Cellular Composition and Sampling of the Transformation Zone

TBS defines a fully *Satisfactory* specimen as containing both squamous cells and endocervical or squamous metaplastic cells (see criteria below). These cellular elements form the microscopic basis for the assumption that the transformation zone has been sampled.

Data in the literature are inconclusive with regard to the endocervical component as a measure of specimen adequacy. Cross-sectional studies have repeatedly demonstrated that smears with endocervical cells have a significantly higher frequency and higher grade of squamous epithelial abnormalities detected than do smears lacking such cells. Furthermore, reviews of positive and negative smears from women with known high-grade squamous intraepithelial lesions (HSILs) and carcinoma have found that positive specimens are more likely than negative ones to have metaplastic squamous cells or both endocervical columnar cells and metaplastic squamous cells. Although compelling, these findings are tempered by observations indicating that specimens without an endocervical component nevertheless often may detect squamous epithelial abnormalities and that, to date, short-term longitudinal studies have demonstrated no increase in the frequency of such lesions on follow-up among women whose entry smears lacked endocervical cells.

The presence of both squamous and endocervical cells does not guarantee adequate sampling of the transformation zone. Conversely, an optimal specimen from a postmenopausal woman may lack endocervical cells because of normal physiologic changes, not poor technique. The clinician ultimately determines what is "adequate sampling" for an individual patient, based on integrating information from the clinical history, visual inspection of the cervix, and the cytopathology report.

Definitions and Criteria for Specimen Adequancy

"Satisfactory for evaluation" indicates that the specimen has all of the following (Figs. 1 and 2):

Appropriate labeling and identifying information
Relevant clinical information
Adequate numbers of well-preserved and well-visualized squamous epithelial cells
An adequate endocervical/transformation zone component (from a patient with a cervix)

Well-preserved and well-visualized squamous epithelial cells should cover more than 10% of the slide surface. An adequate endocervical/transformation zone component should consist, at a minimum, of two clusters of well-preserved endocervical glandular and/or squamous metaplastic cells, with each cluster composed of at least five cells. This definition applies to specimens from both premenopausal and postmenopausal women with a cervix, except in the situation of marked atrophy in which metaplastic and endocervical cells often cannot be distinguished from parabasal-like cells. In cases of marked atrophic changes, the absence of an identifiable endocervical/transformation zone component does not affect the specimen adequacy categorization of a specimen otherwise determined to be "Satisfactory for evaluation."

A specimen is "Satisfactory for evaluation but limited by . . ." if any of the following apply:

Lack of pertinent clinical patient information (age, date of last menstrual period as a minimum; additional information as appropriate)
Partially obscuring blood, inflammation, thick areas, poor fixation, air-drying artifact, contaminant, etc. that precludes interpretation of approximately 50% to 75% of the epithelial cells
Absence of an endocervical/transformation zone component as defined above

"Satisfactory for evaluation but limited by . . ." indicates that the specimen provides useful information; however, interpretation may be compromised. A report of "Satisfactory for evaluation but limited by absence of endocervical/transformation zone component" does not necessarily require a repeat smear. Patient factors such as location of the transformation zone, age, pregnancy, and previous therapy may limit the clinician's ability to obtain an endocervical sample. The ultimate determi-

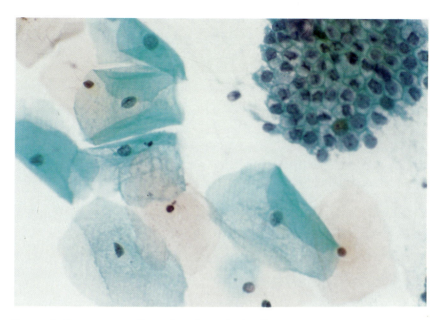

FIGURE 1. Squamous cells and endocervical cells.

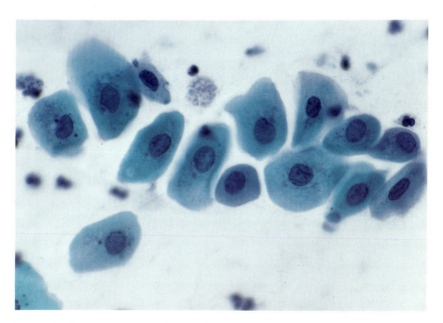

FIGURE 2. Squamous metaplastic cells.

nation of specimen adequacy rests with the clinician, who must correlate the findings described in the cytopathology report with clinical knowledge of the individual patient.

A specimen is "Unsatisfactory for evaluation . . ." if any of the following apply:

Lack of patient identification on the specimen and/or requisition form
A slide that is broken and cannot be repaired
Scant squamous epithelial component (well-preserved and well-visualized squamous epithelial cells covering less than 10% of the slide surface)
Obscuring blood, inflammation, thick areas, poor fixation, air-drying artifact, contaminant, etc. that precludes interpretation of approximately 75% or more of the epithelial cells.

The "Unsatisfactory . . ." designation indicates that the specimen is unreliable for the detection of cervical epithelial abnormalities.

Specimen adequacy is evaluated in all cases.* However, any epithelial abnormality is of paramount importance and must be reported regardless of comprised specimen adequacy. If abnormal cells are detected, the specimen is never categorized as "Unsatisfactory". Such cases may be considered "Satisfactory" or "Satisfactory but limited by . . ." based on the above criteria.†

---

*Most cytotechnologists and cytopathologists incorporate a statement of adequacy in all cervical/vaginal cases. However, a minority viewpoint maintains that "Satisfactory for evaluation" is presumed if no specific reference to adequacy is included in the report.
†A minority view holds that smears containing abnormal cells should automatically be considered "Satisfactory" (since the specimen has accomplished its purpose) and that therefore morphologic criteria for adequacy would not pertain.

Part 2

Descriptive Diagnoses

Definitions, Criteria, and Explanatory Notes

Descriptive Diagnoses

Benign Cellular Changes

Infection

Trichomonas vaginalis
Fungal organisms morphologically consistent with *Candida* spp.
Predominance of coccobacilli consistent with shift in vaginal flora
Bacteria morphologically consistent with *Actinomyces* spp.
Cellular changes associated with Herpes simplex virus
Other*

Reactive Changes

Reactive Cellular Changes Associated With:

Inflammation (includes typical repair)
Atrophy with inflammation ("atrophic vaginitis")
Radiation
Intrauterine contraceptive device (IUD)
Other

Epithelial Cell Abnormalities

Squamous Cell

Atypical squamous cells of undetermined significance (ASCUS): Qualify†
Low-grade squamous intraepithelial lesion (LSIL)
   Encompassing: Human papillomavirus (HPV)*/mild dysplasia/cervical
   intraepithelial neoplasia (CIN) 1
High-grade squamous intraepithelial lesion (HSIL)
   Encompassing: Moderate dysplasia, severe dysplasia, and carcinoma in
   situ/CIN 2 and CIN 3
Squamous cell carcinoma

---

*Cellular changes of HPV cytopathic effect, previously termed "koilocytosis," "koilocytotic atypia," or "condylomatous atypia," are included in the category of LSIL.

†Atypical squamous or glandular cells of undetermined significance should be qualified further, if possible, as to whether a reactive or a neoplastic process is favored.

Glandular Cell

Endometrial cells, cytologically benign, in a postmenopausal woman
Atypical glandular cells of undetermined significance (AGUS): Qualify†
Endocervical adenocarcinoma
Endometrial adenocarcinoma
Extrauterine adenocarcinoma
Adenocarcinoma, NOS

Other Malignant Neoplasms

Specify

Benign Cellular Changes

Infection

Trichomonas vaginalis (Fig. 3):
Criteria
Pear-shaped cyanophilic organism ranging in size from 15 to 30 μm
Nucleus is pale, vesicular, and eccentrically located
Eosinophilic cytoplasmic granules are often evident
Leptothrix may be seen in association with *T. vaginalis*; this finding alone
   is not diagnostic, but suggests the presence of trichomonads.

Fungal Organisms Morphologically Consistent With *Candida* spp. (Fig. 4):
Criteria
Budding yeasts (3–7 μm), pseudohyphae, and true hyphae appear eosino-
   philic to gray-brown with the Papanicolaou stain
Pseudohyphae, formed by elongated budding, show constrictions along
   their length
Fragmented leukocyte nuclei and rouleau formation of squamous epithelial
   cells "speared" by hyphae may be seen.

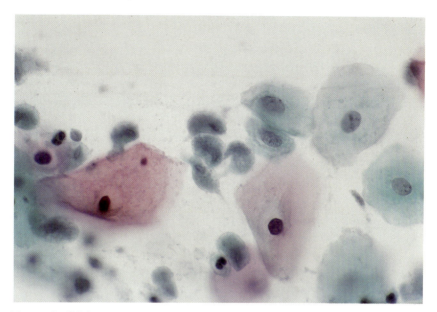

FIGURE 3. *Trichomonas vaginalis.*

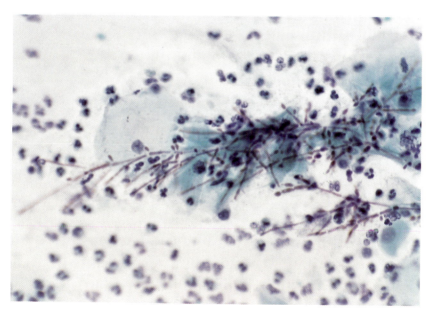

FIGURE 4. Fungal organisms morphologically consistent with *Candida* spp.

Predominance of Coccobacilli Consistent With Shift in Vaginal Flora (Fig. 5):

Criteria

Filmy background of small coccobacilli is evident

Individual squamous cells may be covered by a layer of coccobacilli, particularly along the margin of the cell membrane, forming so-called clue cells

There is a conspicuous absence of lactobacilli.

Bacteria Morphologically Consistent With *Actinomyces* spp. (Fig. 6):

Criteria

Tangled clumps of filamentous organisms with acute angle branching usually are recognizable as "cotton ball" clusters on low power

"Sulfur granules," formed by masses of leukocytes adherent to microcolonies of the organism, with swollen filaments or "clubs" at the periphery, may be identified

An acute inflammatory response with polymorphonuclear leukocytes usually is evident.

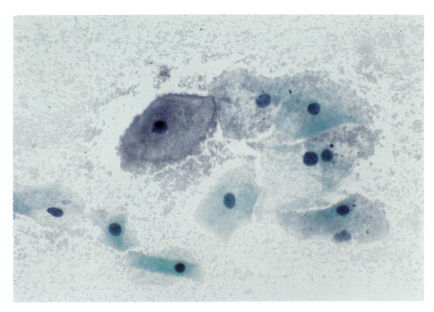

FIGURE 5. Predominance of coccobacilli consistent with shift in vaginal flora.

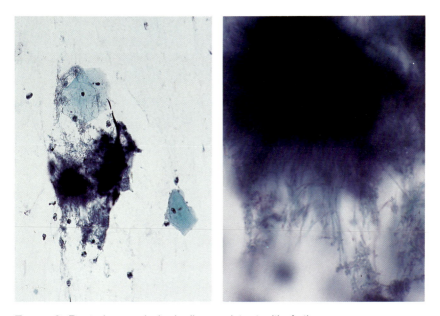

FIGURE 6. Bacteria morphologically consistent with *Actinomyces* spp.

Cellular Changes Associated with Herpes Simplex Virus (Fig. 7):
Criteria

Nuclei have a gelatinous "ground-glass" appearance with enhancement of
the nuclear envelope caused by peripheral margination of chromatin

Dense eosinophilic intranuclear inclusions surrounded by a halo or clear
zone, are variably present

Large multinucleated epithelial cells with molded nuclei are characteristic
but may not always be present; mononucleate cells with the nuclear
features described above also may be diagnostic.

Explanatory Notes and Diagnostic Problems

Lactobacilli consist of a diverse group of *Lactobacillus* spp., which
constitute a major component of the normal vaginal flora. Predominance of
coccobacilli represents a shift in vaginal flora from Lactobacilli to a
polymicrobial process involving several types of obligate and facultative
anaerobic bacteria, including but not limited to *Gardnerella vaginalis* and
Mobiluncus spp. This observation may, in the proper clinical context,
provide supportive evidence for the clinical diagnosis of bacterial vagino-
sis. However, this shift in flora (with or without accompanying clue cells)
is neither specific nor sufficient for that diagnosis.

The diagnosis of *Chlamydia* spp. is not included in TBS because of the
acknowledged low diagnostic accuracy of routine cytology for this organism. More specific detection methods such as culture and enzyme-linked
immunoassay are available.

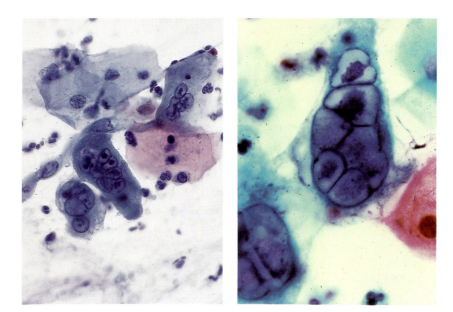

FIGURE 7. Cellular changes associated with Herpes simplex virus.

Reactive Changes

Definition

Reactive cellular changes that are benign in nature, associated with inflammation (includes typical repair), atrophy with inflammation ("atrophic vaginitis"), radiation, an IUD, and other nonspecific causes.

Reactive Cellular Changes Associated With Inflammation (Figs. 8–12):

Criteria

Nuclear enlargement usually is minimal (one and a half to two times the area of a normal intermediate squamous cell nucleus); an exception are endocervical cells, which may show greater nuclear enlargement

Occasional binucleation or multinucleation may be observed

Mild hyperchromasia may be present but the chromatin structure and distribution remain uniformly finely granular

Nuclear degeneration may result in karyopyknosis and karyorrhexis

Nuclear outlines are smooth, rounded, and uniform

Prominent single or multiple nucleoli may be present

The cytoplasm may show polychromasia, vacuolization, or perinuclear halos but without peripheral thickening

In typical repair, any of the above cellular changes may be seen; however, cells occur in flat, monolayer sheets with maintenance of nuclear polarity and typical mitotic figures; single cells with nuclear changes usually are not seen (Fig. 12).

(Figs. 10–12 follow.)

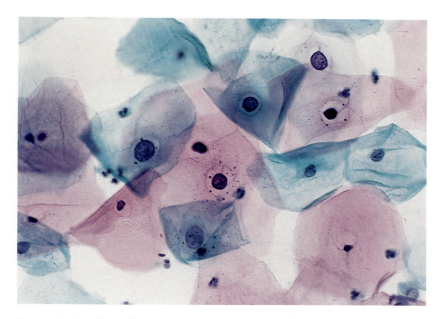

FIGURE 8. Reactive cellular changes—squamous cells.

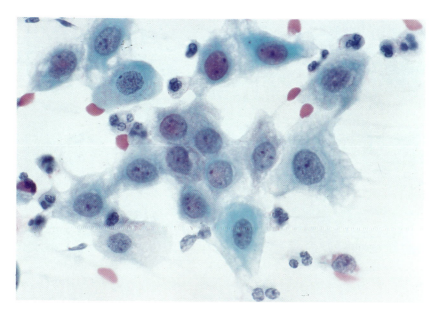

FIGURE 9. Reactive cellular changes—squamous metaplastic cells.

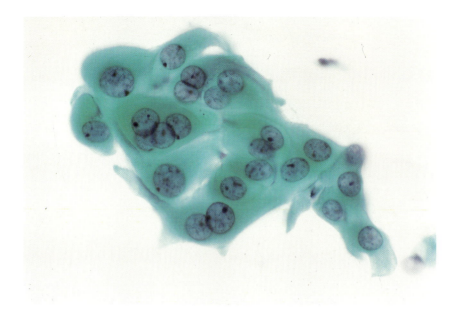

FIGURE 10. Reactive cellular changes—squamous metaplastic cells.

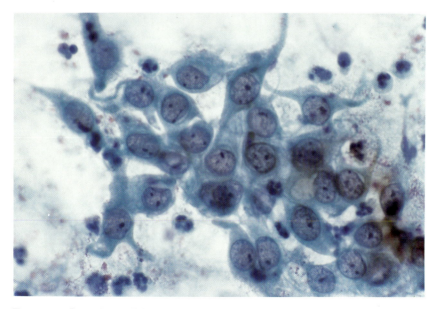

FIGURE 11. Reactive cellular changes—columnar cells.

Reactive Cellular Changes Associated With Atrophy With or Without Inflammation (Fig. 13):

Criteria

There is a generalized nuclear enlargement in atrophic squamous or parabasal-like cells but without significant hyperchromasia

Autolysis may result in naked nuclei

Degenerated orangeophilic or eosinophilic parabasal-like cells with nuclear pyknosis resembling parakeratotic cells may be present

An abundant inflammatory exudate and basophilic granular background that resembles a tumor diathesis may be present

Characteristic basophilic amorphous material (blue blobs) may be seen, which probably reflect degenerated parabasal-like cells

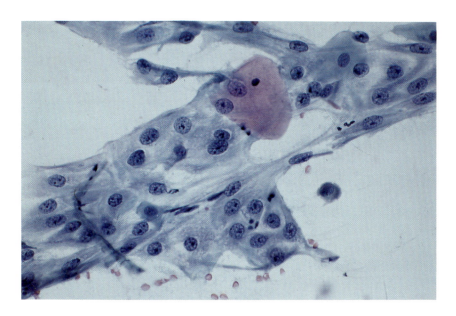

FIGURE 12. Reactive cellular changes—repair.

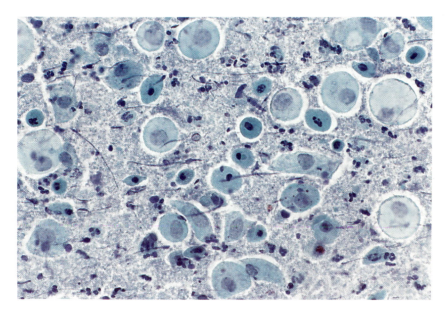

FIGURE 13. Atrophy with inflammation (atrophic vaginitis).

Reactive Cellular Changes Associated With Radiation
(Figs. 14, 15):
Criteria

Cell size is markedly increased without a substantial increase in the nuclear/cytoplasmic ratio

Bizarre cell shapes may occur

Enlarged nuclei may show degenerative changes including nuclear pallor, wrinkling or smudging of the chromatin, and nuclear vacuolization

Nuclei vary in size, with some cell groups having both enlarged and normal-sized nuclei; binucleation or multinucleation is common

Some nuclear hyperchromasia may be present

Prominent single or multiple nucleoli may be seen if a coexisting reparative reaction is present (Fig. 15)

Cytoplasmic vacuolization and/or cytoplasmic polychromatic staining reaction may be seen.

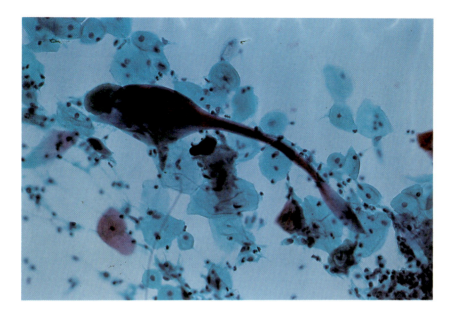

FIGURE 14. Reactive cellular changes associated with radiation.

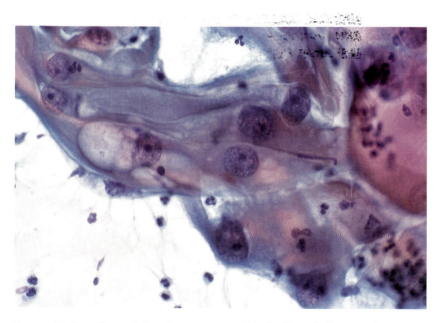

FIGURE 15. Reactive cellular changes associated with radiation repair.

Reactive Cellular Changes Associated With IUD (Figs. 16, 17):
Criteria

Glandular cells occur in small clusters, usually 5 to 15 cells, in a clean
   background (Fig. 16)

Occasional single epithelial cells with increased nuclear size and high
   nuclear/cytoplasmic ratio may be present (Fig. 17)

Nuclear degeneration frequently is evident

Nucleoli may be prominent

The amount of cytoplasm varies and frequently large vacuoles may
   displace the nucleus, creating a signet-ring appearance

Calcifications resembling psammona bodies are variably present.

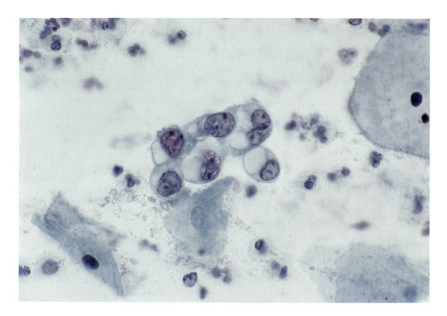

FIGURE 16. Reactive cellular changes associated with IUD.

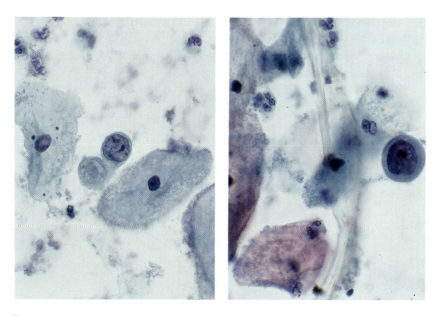

FIGURE 17. Reactive cellular changes associated with IUD.

Explanatory Notes and Diagnostic Problems

This category includes reparative changes or "typical repair," which may involve squamous, squamous metaplastic, or columnar epithelium. The increased nuclear size and prominent nucleoli characteristic of repair may raise concern of a more significant lesion. However, in a reparative process, cells occur in monolayer sheets with nuclei oriented in the same direction, imparting a streaming look to the epithelial fragments. In addition, there is an absence of single cells with nuclear changes. If marked anisonucleosis, irregularities in chromatin distribution, or variation in size and shape of nucleoli are present, so-called atypical repair, the changes should be categorized as atypical squamous or glandular cells of undetermined significance (see Fig. 27, to follow).

A spectrum of morphologic changes may be seen in the context of atrophy. Cellular changes include (1) intermediate-type cells with normochromatic or mildly hyperchromatic nuclei enlarged three to five times the area of a normal atrophic squamous cell nucleus, (2) degeneration resulting in orangeophilic, parakeratotic-like cells with hyperchromatic pyknotic nuclei, (3) monolayer sheets of immature basal-like cells with slightly enlarged nuclei that may be elongated and hyperchromatic, and (4) stripped nuclei resulting from autolysis. Although atrophic squamous cells may demonstrate nuclear enlargement and/or slight hyperchromasia, chromatin distribution and nuclear contours remain uniform. Note that air-drying, a common problem with this type of specimen, may artifactually cause nuclear enlargement. Inflammation, a granular basophilic background, and "blue blobs," thought to represent inspissated mucus or degenerated cells, are variably present.

Acute radiation-induced changes generally disappear several weeks after therapy completion. However, in some patients alterations may persist indefinitely. These chronic changes can include nuclear enlargement, mild hyperchromasia, and persistent polychromatic staining reaction of the cytoplasm. Certain chemotherapeutic agents may produce changes in cervical epithelial cells similar to those seen with acute and chronic radiation effect.

The reactive glandular cell clusters occasionally seen in women with IUDs may represent either endometrial or endocervical columnar cells. They are exfoliated as a result of chronic irritation by the device and may persist for several months after removal of the IUD. Cells may be shed in two patterns: as three-dimensional clusters or singly. The three-dimensional glandular clusters with vacuolated cytoplasm and nuclear changes may closely resemble clusters of cells derived from adenocarcinoma of the endometrium, fallopian tube, or ovary. Single cells with high nuclear/cytoplasmic ratio may mimic a high-grade SIL; however, the morphologic spectrum of abnormalities usually present with true precursor lesions is absent. In general, the diagnosis of adenocarcinoma should be made only with caution in the presence of an IUD. If there is any doubt as to the significance of the cellular abnormalities, the cytopathologist should consider recommending removal of the IUD followed by repeat smear.

Epithelial Cell Abnormalities

Squamous Cell

Atypical Squamous Cells of Undetermined Significance (ASCUS) (Figs. 18–24; 26–31):

Definition

Cellular abnormalities that are more marked than those attributable to reactive changes but that quantitatively or qualitatively fall short of a definitive diagnosis of squamous intraepithelial lesion (SIL). Because the cellular changes in the ASCUS category may reflect an exuberant benign change or a potentially serious lesion, which cannot be unequivocally classified, they are interpreted as being of undetermined significance.

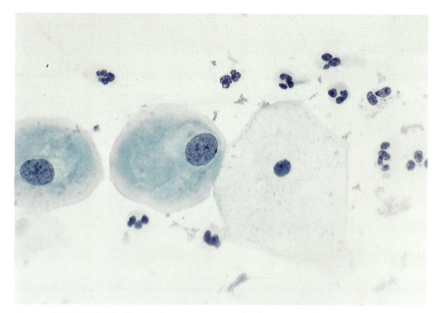

FIGURE 18. ASCUS: Atypical squamous cells, favor reactive.

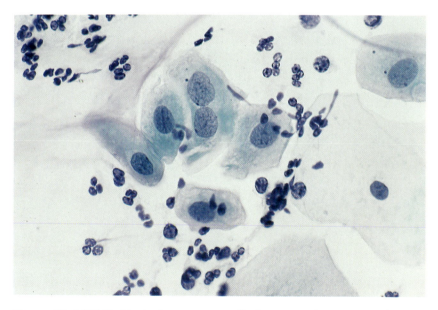

FIGURE 19. ASCUS: Atypical squamous cells, favor reactive.

Criteria

Nuclear enlargement is two and a half to three times that of a normal intermediate squamous cell nucleus with a slight increase in the nuclear/cytoplasmic ratio

Variation in nuclear size and shape, and binucleation, may be observed

Mild hyperchromasia may be present, but the chromatin remains evenly distributed without granularity

Nuclear outlines usually are smooth and regular; very limited irregularity may be observed.

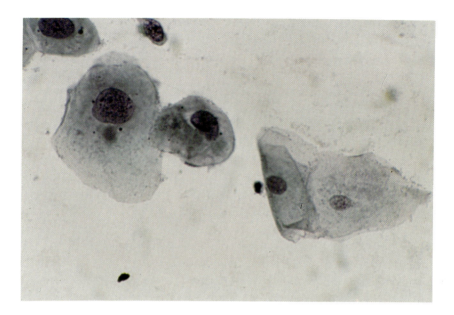

FIGURE 20. ASCUS.

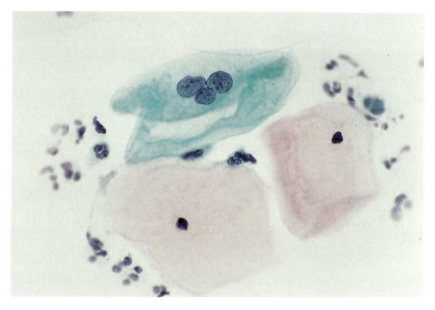

FIGURE 21. ASCUS.

Explanatory Notes and Diagnostic Problems

ASCUS is a diagnosis of exclusion for cytopathologic findings that are not sufficiently clear-cut to permit a more specific diagnosis. Despite efforts to provide specific criteria for what constitutes ASCUS, the use of this term by various pathologists may differ. However, as a general guide the frequency of ASCUS diagnoses should not exceed 2–3 times the rate of SIL. For example, if the frequency of SIL in a laboratory practice is 2%, the frequency of ASCUS should be less than or equal to 6%.

ASCUS is not synonymous with previously used terms such as "atypia," "benign atypia," "inflammatory atypia," or "reactive atypia," which had included lesions currently classified in TBS as "reactive cellular changes" (see above). Cellular abnormalities in the ASCUS category may be related to a number of etiologic factors but a definitive cause cannot be determined on the basis of the cytologic findings. Exuberant epithelial reactions to inflammation and repair, and nondiagnostic cellular changes predating or accompanying an intraepithelial lesion may have similar cytologic characteristics. Sparsity of abnormal cells and/or artifacts, such as air-drying, which preclude optimal visualization of the cellular material, may contribute to the diagnostic difficulty.

Most often, ASCUS involves nuclear enlargement in squamous cells with mature, superficial/intermediate-type cytoplasm (see Figs. 18–20 earlier). The differential diagnosis is between a benign change in reaction to a stimulus versus a LSIL.

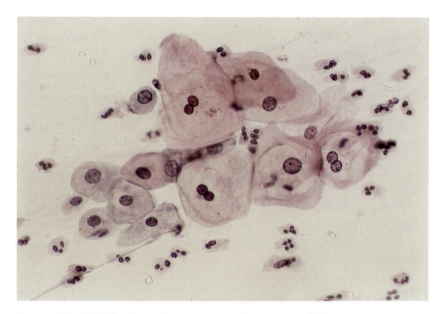

FIGURE 22. ASCUS: Atypical squamous cells, possibly LSIL.

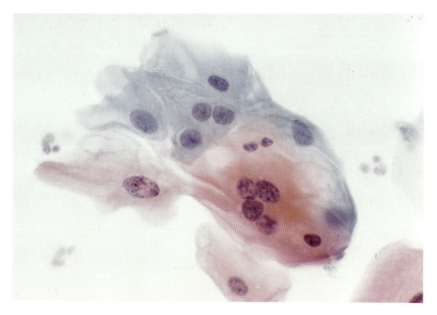

FIGURE 23. ASCUS: Atypical squamous cells, possibly LSIL.

Changes diagnostic of HPV cytopathic effects—well-defined, optically clear, perinuclear cavity associated with a peripheral rim of thickened cytoplasm as well as nuclear alterations—are classified as LSIL. Cells with some but not all of these features, which are suggestive of HPV cytopathic effects, are included in the ASCUS category (see Figs. 21–24). Note that cytoplasmic vacuolization alone, without any nuclear atypia, is considered a benign cellular change and should not be classified as LSIL or ASCUS (Fig. 25).

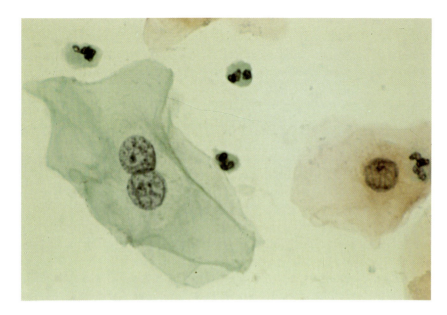

FIGURE 24. ASCUS: Atypical squamous cells, possibly LSIL.

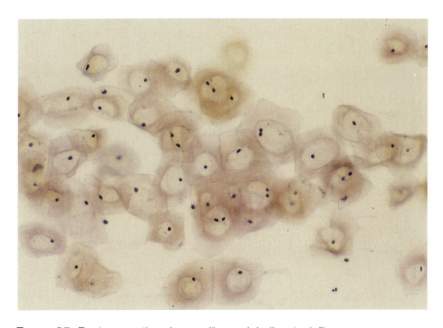

FIGURE 25. Benign reactive change ("pseudokoilocytosis").

Whereas in most cases of ASCUS the cells have mature-appearing cytoplasm, similar changes also may occur in less mature squamous metaplastic cells (so-called atypical metaplasia). Nuclear enlargement approximates one and a half to two times the area of a normal squamous metaplastic nucleus, or three times the area of a normal squamous intermediate-cell nucleus (Fig. 26). In this circumstance, the differential diagnosis is between reactive metaplasia versus a HSIL. LSIL is not a consideration.

Marked cellular changes involving tissue fragments, or sheets of immature squamous cells, so-called atypical repair, also are included in the ASCUS cateogry but present a different cytologic picture. In "typical" repair, cells occur primarily in monolayer sheets and syncytia and contain prominent nucleoli (see Fig. 12 earlier). However, nuclear piling, significant anisonucleosis, and irregularities in chromatin distribution that exceed changes seen in "typical" repair are considered ASCUS (Fig. 27). The differential diagnosis is between an exuberant reparative process versus carcinoma. Atypical reparative reactions, however, lack both a tumor diathesis and the many isolated abnormal cells that are features of squamous cell carcinoma (see below).

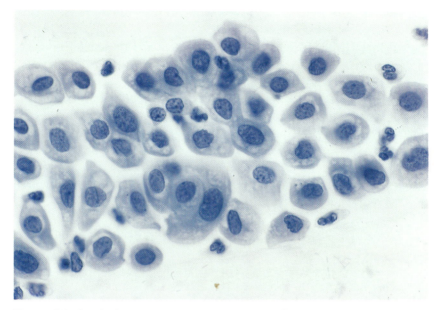

FIGURE 26. Atypical squamous metaplastic cells of undetermined significance.

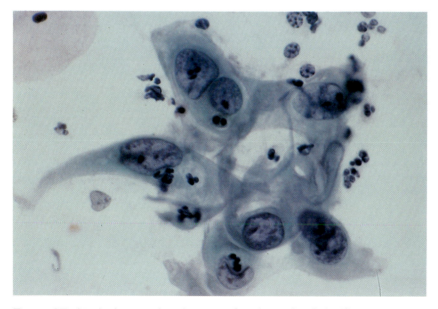

FIGURE 27. Atypical reparative changes of undetermined significance.

A spectrum of benign reactive morphologic changes may be seen in the setting of atrophy (see above). Occasionally these changes become so marked that HSIL or squamous carcinoma cannot be excluded (Figs. 28,29). A diagnosis of ASCUS associated with atrophy should be considered if cells demonstrate (1) both nuclear enlargement (at least two times normal) and significant hyperchromasia, (2) irregularities in nuclear contour or chromatin distribution, or (3) marked pleomorphism in the form of tadpole or spindle cells. A short course of estrogen therapy followed by a repeat smear may be useful to establish a definitive diagnosis. Benign changes caused by atrophy will resolve after estrogen stimulation; atypical changes resulting from a significant precancerous lesion will persist and be detected more easily in a background of mature cells.

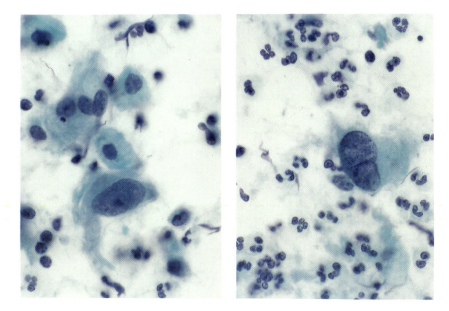

FIGURE 28. ASCUS: Atypical squamous cells associated with atrophy.

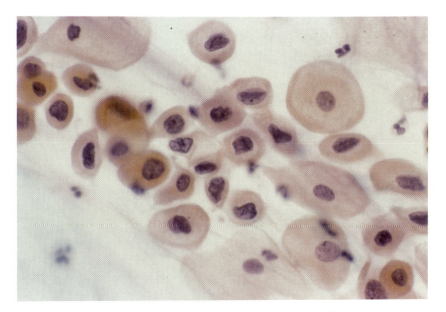

FIGURE 29. ASCUS: Atypical squamous cells associated with atrophy.

Hyperkeratosis, parakeratosis, and dyskeratosis are descriptors that have been used inconsistently in the past and are not included in TBS terminology. The classification of cellular changes previously termed "dyskeratosis," "hyperkeratosis," and "parakeratosis" depends on the cytoplasmic and nuclear alterations present. Anucleate, but otherwise unremarkable mature polygonal squamous cells, so-called hyperkeratosis, may indicate a benign reactive cellular change. Alternatively, inadvertent contamination of the specimen with vulvar material may introduce anucleate squamous cells on the smear. Miniature polygonal squamous cells with dense, orangeophilic, or eosinophilic cytoplasm and small pyknotic nuclei, so-called parakeratosis, usually represent a benign reactive change and should not be considered an epithelial cell abnormality. However, cells shed singly or in three-dimensional clusters that demonstrate cellular pleomorphism—caudate or elongate shapes—and/or increased nuclear size or chromasia should be categorized as ASCUS or SIL depending on the degree of the cellular abnormalities (Figs. 30,31). Such changes have previously been termed "dyskeratosis" or "atypical parakeratosis."

In each of the diagnostic dilemmas discussed above, the cytopathologist must consider the summation of the quantity and severity of the morphologic abnormalities in the context of the clinical information available. Often the diagnosis of ASCUS may be qualified to indicate whether a reactive process or SIL is considered more likely. Communicating the cytopathologist's degree of concern may assist the clinician in determining patient management.

The available data indicate that for many specimens demonstrating ASCUS, patients do not have a significant lesion, and follow-up smears or colposcopic biopsies are normal. In a proportion of patients, however, the abnormality will persist and in a significant number of these, further evaluation will detect a squamous intraepithelial lesion. Conclusions concerning the behavior and management of these lesions await properly controlled clinical trials in which the criteria for ASCUS are carefully defined.

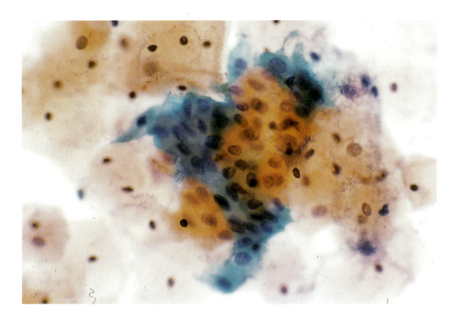

Figure 30. ASCUS: Atypical squamous cells, favor LSIL ("atypical parakeratosis").

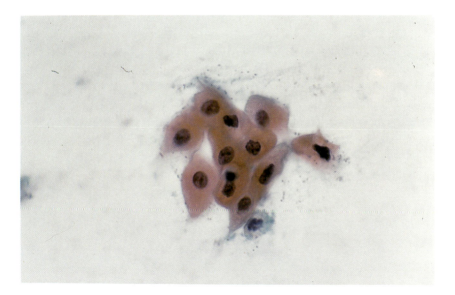

Figure 31. ASCUS: Atypical squamous cells, favor LSIL ("atypical parakeratosis").

Squamous Intraepithelial Lesion (SIL)
Definition
Squamous intraepithelial lesion encompasses a spectrum of noninvasive cervical epithelial abnormalities traditionally classified as flat condyloma, dysplasia/carcinoma in situ, and CIN. In TBS, the spectrum is divided into low-grade and high-grade lesions. Low-grade lesions encompass the cellular changes associated with HPV cytopathic effect (so-called koilocytotic atypia) and mild dysplasia/CIN 1. High-grade lesions encompass moderate dysplasia, severe dysplasia, and carcinoma in situ/CIN 2,3.

LSIL (Figs. 32–35):
Criteria
Cells occur singly or in sheets

Nuclear abnormalities are generally confined to cells with "mature" or superficial-type cytoplasm

Nuclear enlargement is at least three times the area of normal intermediate nuclei, resulting in an increased nuclear/cytoplasmic ratio

Moderate variation in nuclear size and shape is evident

Binucleation or multinucleation often is present

Hyperchromasia is present and the chromatin is uniformly distributed; alternatively, the chromatin may appear degenerated or smudged if associated with the cytopathic changes of HPV

Nucleoli are rarely present, or inconspicuous if present

Nuclear membranes are either clearly visible with slight irregularities or may be completely inapparent when the chromatin is smudged

Distinct cell borders are present

Cells that demonstrate a well-defined, optically clear perinuclear cavity and a peripheral dense rim of cytoplasm must also show the above nuclear abnormalities to be diagnostic of LSIL (Fig. 32); perinuclear halos in the *absence of nuclear abnormalities* do not qualify for the diagnosis (see Fig. 25 earlier).

(Figs. 34–35 follow.)

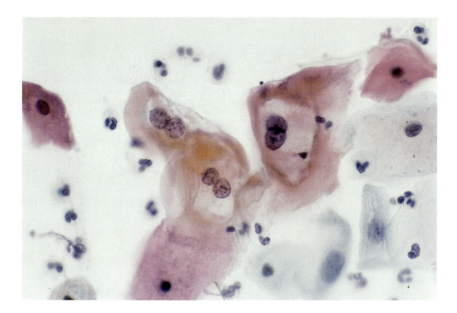

FIGURE 32. LSIL.

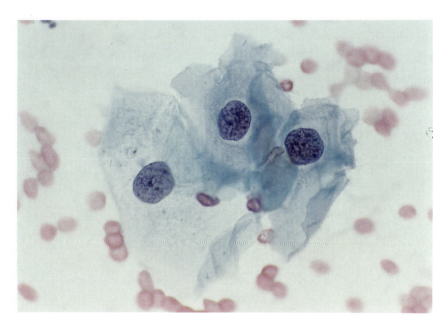

FIGURE 33. LSIL.

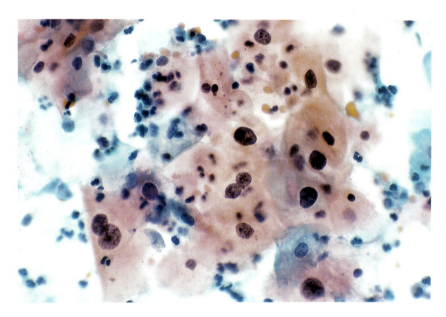

FIGURE 34. LSIL.

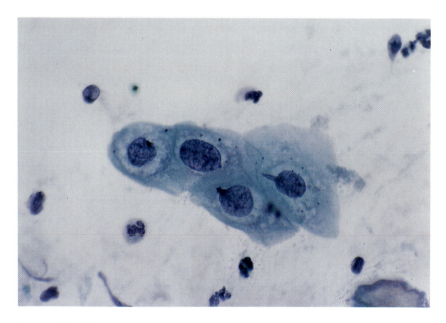

FIGURE 35. LSIL.

HSIL (Figs. 36–43):

Criteria

Cells usually occur singly, in sheets, or in syncytial-like aggregates

Nuclear abnormalities occur predominantly in squamous cells with "immature," lacy, and delicate or dense metaplastic cytoplasm; occasionally the cytoplasm is "mature" and densely keratinized

Nuclear enlargement is in the range of that seen in LSIL but the cytoplasmic area is decreased, leading to a marked increase in the nuclear/cytoplasmic ratio; in cells with very high nuclear/cytoplasmic ratios, the nuclear enlargement actually may be less than that in LSIL

Overall, HSIL cell size is smaller than in LSIL

Hyperchromasia is evident; chromatin may be finely or coarsely granular with an even distribution

Nucleoli are generally absent

Nuclear outlines are irregular.

(Figs. 38–43 follow.)

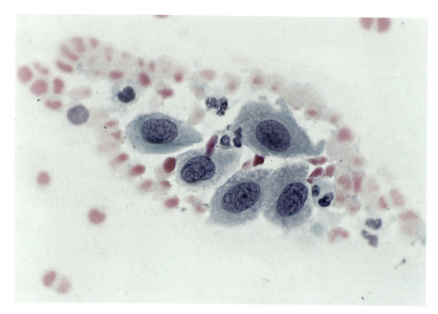

FIGURE 36. HSIL.

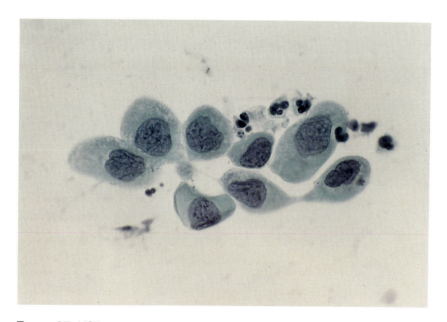

FIGURE 37. HSIL.

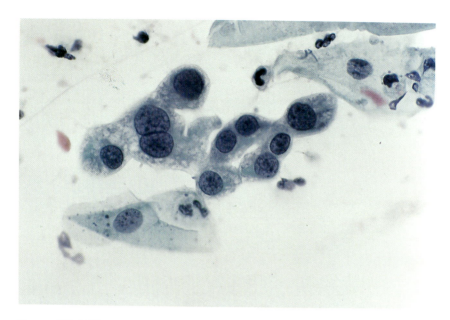

Figure 38. HSIL.

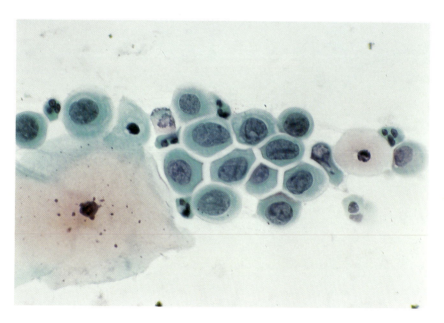

Figure 39. HSIL.

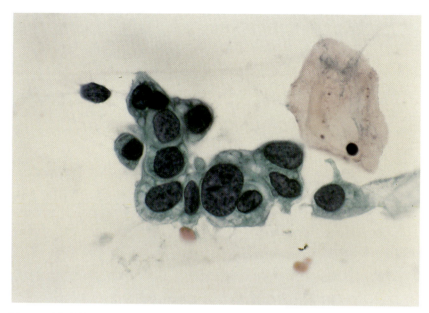

FIGURE 40. HSIL.

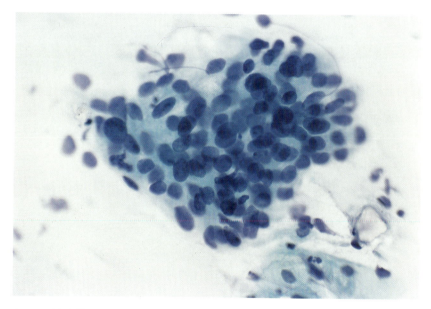

FIGURE 41. HSIL—syncytial-like group.

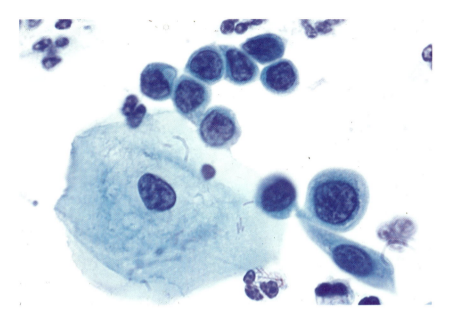

FIGURE 42. HSIL.

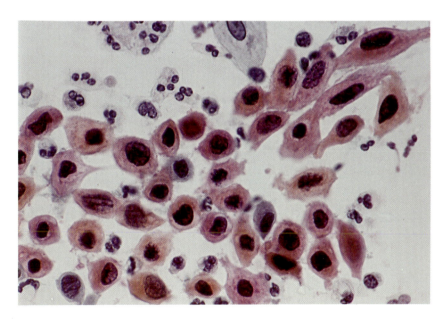

FIGURE 43. HSIL.

Explanatory Notes and Diagnostic Problems

The rationale for introducing the term "squamous intraepithelial lesion" to replace dysplasia/carcinoma in situ (CIS) and cervical intraepithelial neoplasia is based on the observations that most mild dysplasia/CIN 1 regress and approximately half of cases classified as moderate dysplasia/ CIN 2 do not progress. Even severe dysplasia-CIS/CIN 3 does not invariably progress to invasive carcinoma. Although as a group high-grade lesions are more likely to persist or progress than low-grade lesions, the behavior in an individual patient is unpredictable. The term "lesion" rather than "neoplasia" is used to convey the uncertain biologic potential in an individual patient.

The spectrum of cytologic abnormalities in this group is subdivided into two categories as opposed to three or four for several reasons: (1) previous studies have reported low inter- and intraobserver reproducibility with conventional three- and four-grade classification systems, (2) in the current management of HSILs in the United States, nuances of lesion grade are not relevant, (3) accumulated data from natural history studies comparing low- and high-grade lesions imply differences between low- and high-grade intraepithelial lesions, although the biologic behavior of an individual abnormality, whether high or low grade, cannot be predicted. It must be emphasized that cervical cytology is used for screening. The subsequent management of a cytologic diagnosis of LSIL may include follow-up with smears or a directed biopsy. HSIL should be evaluated by colposcopy and directed biopsy. Management should focus on preventing invasive carcinoma by the most conservative means possible.

Mounting evidence over the past 10 years indicates that HPV is a critical factor in the pathogenesis of cervical squamous cell carcinoma. In addition, HPV DNA can be detected by molecular techniques in the vast majority of SILs regardless of the presence of cellular changes of HPV-related cytopathic effect. Therefore, the presence of such morphologic changes does not add substantively to the diagnosis and does not need to be appended to the diagnosis of SIL.

Half to nearly three quarters of invasive cervical cancers contain certain HPV types; these viruses have been referred to as "high-risk" HPVs. High-risk HPVs are associated with both low- and high-grade SIL, but are observed with significantly greater frequency in the high-grade group. Individual cellular features within the morphologic continuum cannot be correlated consistently with HPV DNA types.

Several recent studies have demonstrated that the morphologic criteria for distinguishing "koilocytosis" from CIN 1 vary between investigators and lack reproducibility. In addition, both lesions share similar HPV types and their clinical behavior is similar, thus supporting the inclusion of these lesions in a single category.

Accordingly, in TBS, LSIL encompasses cellular changes associated with HPV, previously designated "koilocytosis," as well as CIN 1. The inclusion of cellular changes of HPV in the category of LSIL requires that the diagnosis be based on strict criteria to avoid overinterpretation and unnecessary treatment of women for nonspecific morphologic changes. Overdiagnosis of cellular changes of HPV is a significant problem, in large part because of interpretation of any cytoplasmic halo without accompanying atypical nuclear features as "koilocytosis" and the use of "nonclassic" cytologic signs of condyloma. Specimens with subtle changes that fall short of definitive SIL are categorized as "atypical squamous cells of undetermined significance" (see Figs. 21–24 earlier). Terms such as "koilocytosis," "koilocytotic atypia," and "condylomatous atypia" are not included in TBS terminology.

Another diagnostic problem is the difficulty in categorizing lesions with intermediate features into low or high grade. Although occasional "borderline" cases occur, most of these can be classified as either LSIL or HSIL. LSIL is characterized by nuclear enlargement at least three times the size of a normal intermediate cell nucleus. Although the nucleus is hyperchromatic, the chromatin is distributed uniformly or it may appear degenerated and smudged if associated with cellular changes of HPV. Features that favor a high-grade lesion include increased numbers of abnormal cells, higher nuclear/cytoplasmic ratios, greater irregularities in the outline of the nuclear envelope, coarsening of nuclear chromatin, and chromatin clumping. The appearance of the cytoplasm also may assist in determining whether a "borderline" case is low- or high-grade SIL: LSIL typically involves squamous cells with "mature," intermediate, or superficial-type cytoplasm with well-defined polygonal cell borders. Cells of an HSIL have a more immature type of cytoplasm, either lacy and delicate or dense/metaplastic, with rounded cell borders. Overall, cell size is smaller in HSIL as compared with LSIL. When it is not possible to grade a SIL as low or high, a diagnosis of "SIL, grade cannot be determined" is appropriate.

Although most HSILs are characterized by cells with a high nuclear/cytoplasmic ratio, some high-grade lesions are composed of cells with more abundant but abnormally keratinized cytoplasm (see Fig. 43 earlier). These cells may be shed singly or in dense clusters and have enlarged hyperchromatic nuclei, often with smudged chromatin. In addition, there is variation in nuclear size (anisokaryosis) and cellular shape (including elongate/spindle and caudate/tadpole cells). In contrast to invasive squamous carcinoma, nucleoli and a tumor diathesis are absent. Such lesions have been previously termed "atypical condyloma," "keratinizing dysplasia," and "pleomorphic dysplasia." At times, these keratinized lesions may be indistinguishable from an invasive carcinoma, especially in samples with relatively scant numbers of abnormal cells. In these instances, an explanatory note may be appended to indicate that the differential diagnosis includes an invasive squamous cell carcinoma.

Although vaginal squamous intraepithelial lesions also are designated LSIL and HSIL, the cytologic features and behavior of these lesions are not as well understood as their cervical counterparts. Histologic confirmation of these lesions is therefore important.

Squamous Cell Carcinoma
Definition
A malignant invasive tumor composed of squamous cells.

The Bethesda System does not subdivide squamous cell carcinoma; however, for purposes of outlining criteria, nonkeratinizing and keratinizing tumors are described separately.

Nonkeratinizing Squamous Cell Carcinoma (Fig. 44):
Criteria
Cells occur singly or in syncytial-like aggregates
Cells display all the features of HSIL but in addition contain prominent
   macronucleoli and markedly irregular distribution of chromatin, including coarse chromatin clumping and parachromatin clearing
An associated tumor diathesis consisting of necrotic debris and old blood
   often is present.

Keratinizing Squamous Cell Carcinoma (Fig. 45):
Criteria
Cells occur singly, less commonly in aggregates
Marked variation in cellular size and shape is seen with caudate and spindle
   cells that frequently contain dense orangeophilic cytoplasm
Nuclei also vary markedly in size and configuration, with numerous dense
   opaque nuclear forms
Chromatin, when discernible, is coarsely granular and irregularly distributed with parachromatin clearing
Macronuclei may be seen but are less common than in nonkeratinizing
   squamous cell carcinoma
A tumor diathesis may be present.

Explanatory Notes and Diagnostic Problems
Invasive squamous cell carcinoma is the most common malignant neoplasm of the uterine cervix. Previous classifications have divided squamous carcinoma into keratinizing, nonkeratinizing, and small cell types. Historically, small cell carcinoma comprised a heterogeneous group of neoplasms, including poorly differentiated squamous cell carcinoma, as well as tumors demonstrating neuroendocrine features when evaluated by electron microscopic or immunohistochemical techniques. In TBS, poorly differentiated carcinomas with evidence of squamous differentiation are included in the squamous cell carcinoma category. In contrast, tumors that are undifferentiated by light microscopy or those that demonstrate neuroendocrine features are classified under "other malignant neoplasms" (Fig. 61).

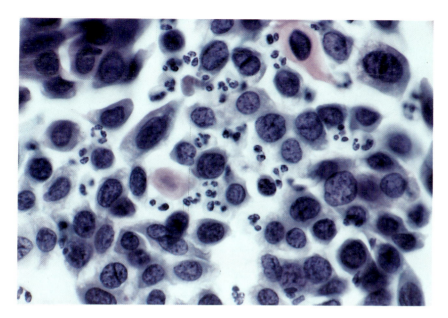

FIGURE 44. Squamous cell carcinoma—nonkeratinizing.

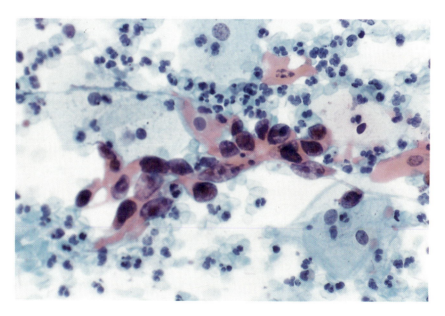

FIGURE 45. Squamous cell carcinoma—keratinizing.

Glandular Cell

Endometrial Cells, Cytologically Benign, in a Postmenopausal Woman

Benign Endometrial Epithelial Cells (Fig. 46):
Criteria
Cells occur in small clusters and less commonly as single cells

A sheet-like pattern is seen when endometrial cells are obtained directly from the lower uterine segment or endometrial cavity

Small, round nuclei approximate the size of normal intermediate squamous cell nuclei

Small or inconspicuous nucleoli are typical

Cell borders are ill-defined and cytoplasm is scant, basophilic, and sometimes vacuolated.

Benign Endometrial Stromal Cells (Fig. 47):
Criteria
Deep stromal cells may vary from round to spindle-shaped, with small, oval nuclei and scant cytoplasm

Superficial stromal cells with decidual changes have abundant foamy cytoplasm and may be difficult to distinguish from endometrial epithelial cells and histiocytes.

Explanatory Notes and Diagnostic Problems
The appearance of endometrial cells depends on the time in the menstrual cycle, sampling technique, and cell type. Spontaneously exfoliated endometrial cells may appear in vaginal smears, cervical scrapings, and endocervical brushings during the proliferative phase of the menstrual cycle. During the 6th to 10th day of the cycle, endometrial cells appear as double-contoured masses that consist of inner stromal cells and outer epithelial cells. The presence of endometrial cells, epithelial or stromal, even when normal in appearance, in a postmenopausal woman not on hormonal therapy must be explained. Such endometrial cells may be associated with vigorous sampling of the lower uterine segment, endometrial polyps, hormonal therapy, IUD, endometrial hyperplasia, or endometrial carcinoma.

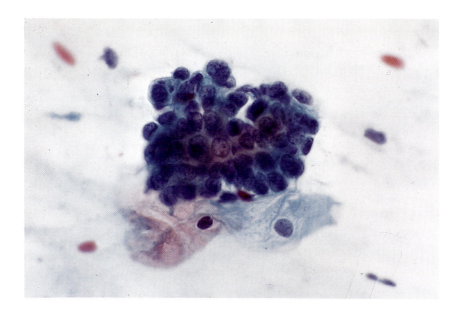

FIGURE 46. Endometrial epithelial cells.

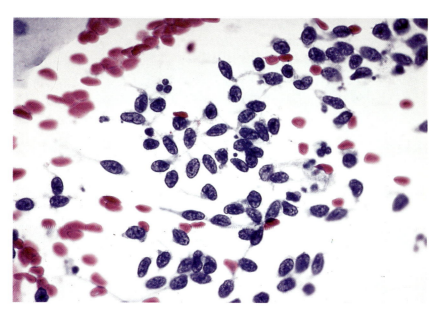

FIGURE 47. Endometrial stromal cells.

Atypical Glandular Cells of Undetermined Significance (AGUS)
Definition
Cells showing either endometrial or endocervical differentiation display-
ing nuclear atypia that exceeds obvious reactive or reparative changes but
lack unequivocal features of invasive adenocarcinoma.

Atypical Endometrial Cells of Undetermined Significance
(Fig. 48):
Criteria
Cells occur in small groups, usually 5 to 10 cells per group
Nuclei are slightly enlarged
Slight hyperchromasia may be seen
Small nucleoli may be present
Cell borders are ill-defined
Compared with endocervical cells, these cells have scant cytoplasm, which
   occasionally is vacuolated.

Atypical Endocervical Cells, Favor Reactive (Fig. 49):
Criteria
Cells occur in sheets and strips with minor degrees of nuclear overlap
Nuclear enlargement, up to three to five times the area of normal
   endocervical nuclei, may be seen
Mild variation in nuclear size and shape occurs
Slight hyperchromasia frequently is evident
Nucleoli often are present
Abundant cytoplasm and distinct cell borders often are discernible.

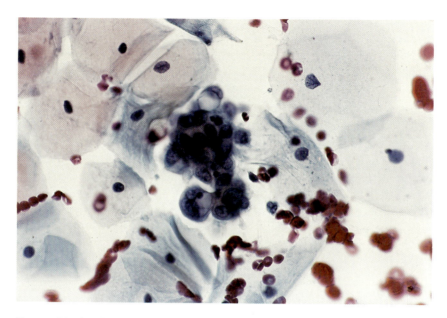

FIGURE 48. Atypical endometrial cells of undetermined significance.

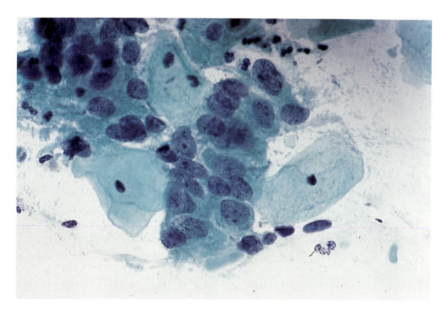

FIGURE 49. Atypical endocervical cells, favor reactive.

Atypical Endocervical Cells, Probably Neoplastic (Figs. 50–53):
Criteria

Abnormal cells occur in sheets, strips and rosettes with nuclear crowding and overlap; when in sheets, a honeycomb pattern is lost because of an increase in the nuclear/cytoplasmic ratio, diminished cytoplasm, and ill-defined cell borders

A palisading nuclear arrangement with nuclei protruding from the periphery of cell clusters (feathering) is a characteristic feature

Nuclear enlargement, elongation, and stratification are evident in most cases

Variation in nuclear size and shape occurs

Hyperchromasia associated with chromatin that is finely to moderately granular usually is evident

Nucleoli are small or inconspicuous

Mitotic figures may be seen.

(Figs. 52–53 follow.)

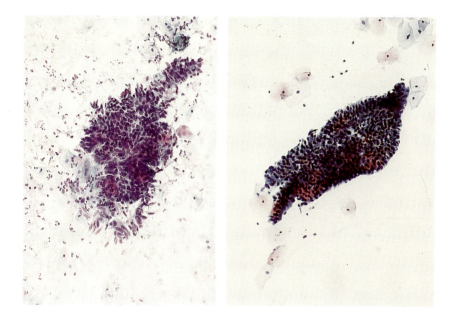

FIGURE 50. Atypical endocervical cells, probably neoplastic [adenocarcinoma in situ (AIS)] (low power).

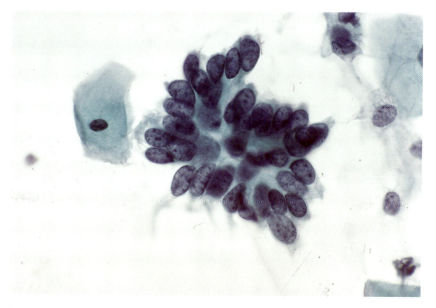

FIGURE 51. Atypical endocervical cells, probably neoplastic (AIS).

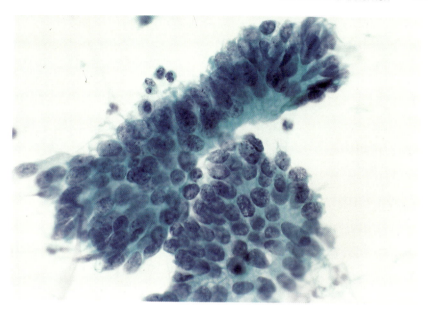

FIGURE 52. Atypical endocervical cells, probably neoplastic (AIS).

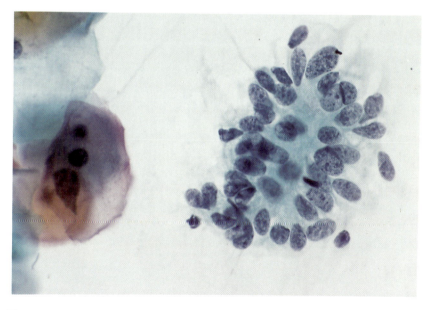

FIGURE 53. Atypical endocervical cells, probably neoplastic (AIS).

Explanatory Notes and Diagnostic Problems

The diagnosis of AGUS should be qualified, if possible, to indicate whether the cells are thought to be of endocervical or endometrial origin. If the origin of the glandular cells cannot be determined, the diagnosis of AGUS is used. Atypical endocervical cells may be subclassified further according to whether a reactive or neoplastic process is favored. If this distinction cannot be made, the diagnosis of "atypical endocervical cells of undetermined significance" is used (Fig. 54). In contrast, criteria for separating atypical endometrial cells into those most likely reflecting a reactive versus a neoplastic process are not well defined and therefore this category is not further subdivided.

The distinction of cytologically benign versus atypical endometrial cells is based primarily on the criterion of slightly increased nuclear size. The presence of atypical endometrial cells, like their cytologically bland counterparts (see above), may be associated with the presence of endometrial polyps, chronic endometritis, IUD, endometrial hyperplasia, or endometrial carcinoma.

The category of atypical endocervical cells encompasses a broad morphologic spectrum of changes that exceed reactive change but fall short of frankly invasive adenocarcinoma. Accordingly, lesions in this category can range from benign, but atypical-appearing reactive processes, to adenocarcinoma in situ (AIS).

As with squamous cells, there are a variety of reactive and reparative changes that can occur in glandular cells. These cytologic alterations are sufficiently well defined so as not to be included in the AGUS category but rather in the category of reactive cellular changes. Benign reactive endocervical cells display the honeycomb sheet-like arrangement of normal endocervical cells with abundant cytoplasm, well-defined cell borders, and minimal nuclear overlap. The nuclei retain the round to oval configuration of normal endocervical cells but are enlarged, sometimes several times that of normal. Nuclear contour is smooth or slightly irregular. Nuclei may be slightly hyperchromatic but they retain a finely granular chromatin pattern. Multinucleated forms also occur. Nucleoli frequently are seen in cases of inflammation and repair.

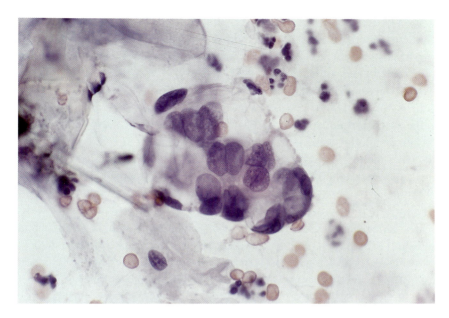

FIGURE 54. Atypical endocervical cells of undetermined significance.

Reactive but atypical-appearing endocervical cells may occur with cervicitis and also may coexist with an overlying SIL. Microglandular hyperplasia and Arias–Stella change of the endocervical glands also can give rise to these atypical cells.

Endocervical cells may be ciliated. Ciliated pseudostratified columnar cells occurring in clusters represent tubal metaplasia. The nuclei of these cells are enlarged and hyperchromatic and may resemble AIS (Figs. 55,56). Although there is overlap of some cytologic features with AIS and invasive adenocarcinoma, the nuclei in tubal metaplasia tend to be round or oval and display more finely granular, evenly dispersed chromatin. In addition, feathered edges, rosette formation, and mitoses are uncommon. The most helpful criterion is the presence of cilia.

The natural history and outcome of glandular intraepithelial lesions that fall short of AIS are not known. HPV DNA has been demonstrated in most invasive endocervical adenocarcinomas and AIS. A much lower detection rate of HPV DNA in atypical glandular lesions suggests that lesions that fall short of AIS may be unrelated to cervical carcinogenesis. Further study of this category is therefore necessary to define more clearly the morphologic features and behavior of these lesions.

Recent studies have begun to delineate the features of AIS (see Criteria for atypical endocervical cells, probably neoplastic). Although at times a diagnosis of AIS can be made with a certain degree of assurance, frequently it is extremely difficult to distinguish AIS from tubal metaplasia, an exuberant reactive process, or for that matter from invasive adenocarcinoma. Additional studies therefore are needed to validate the reproducibility of the criteria of AIS. In TBS, specimens with features of AIS are classified within the category of atypical endocervical cells, probably neoplastic.

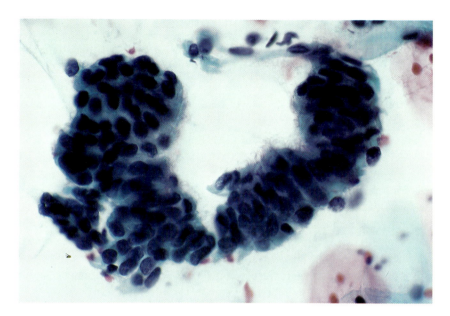

FIGURE 55. Tubal metaplasia.

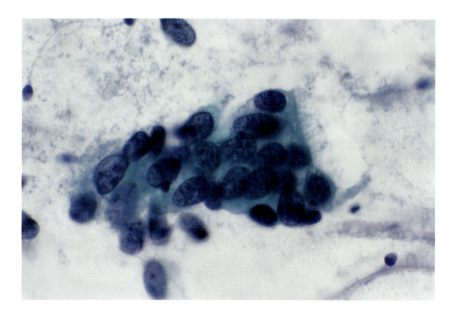

FIGURE 56. Tubal metaplasia.

Endocervical Adenocarcinoma (Fig. 57):
Definition
A malignant invasive neoplasm composed of endocervical-type cells.

Criteria
Cytologic criteria include those outlined for atypical endocervical cells,
   probably neoplastic (see above)
Single cells, two-dimensional sheets, or clusters may be seen
Enlarged nuclei demonstrate irregular chromatin distribution and para-
   chromatin clearing
Macronucleoli may be present
A necrotic tumor diathesis may be evident
Columnar cell shape may be retained with eosinophilic or cyanophilic
   cytoplasm
Abnormal squamous cells additionally may be present, representing either
   a coexisting squamous lesion or the squamous component of an
   adenocarcinoma showing partial squamous differentiation

Explanatory Notes and Diagnostic Problems
Most invasive cervical adenocarcinomas are preceded by precursor lesions
that have been designated AIS. As noted above, lesions thought to reflect
AIS are reported as "atypical endocervical cells, probably neoplastic."
However, there is considerable morphologic overlap between this category
and invasive adenocarcinoma. Criteria indicating invasion such as tumor
diathesis and macronucleoli may be absent in most well-differentiated,
early adenocarcinomas. Therefore, the differentiation of "atypical endocervical cells, probably neoplastic" from invasive carcinoma often requires
histologic evaluation. In the presence of a tumor diathesis, nuclear clearing
with uneven distribution of chromatin or macronucleoli, an invasive
adenocarcinoma should be strongly considered.
   A wide variety of histologic types of adenocarcinoma besides the typical
mucinous endocervical type occur in the endocervix. These include
endometrioid, intestinal, clear cell, and serous neoplasms.

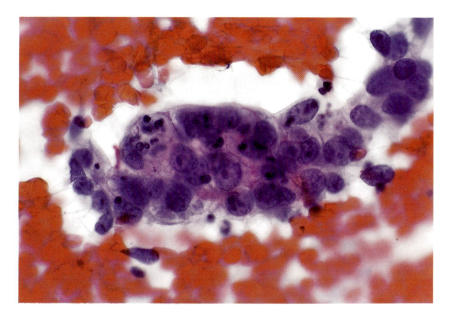

FIGURE 57. Endocervical adenocarcinoma.

Endometrial Adenocarcinoma (Fig. 58):
Definition
A malignant neoplasm composed of endometrial-type cells. The cytologic appearance varies with the degree of differentiation.

Criteria
Cells typically occur singly or in small, loose clusters
In well-differentiated tumors, nuclei may be only slightly increased in size, becoming larger with increasing grade of tumor
Variation in nuclear size and loss of nuclear polarity are evident
Particularly in higher grade tumors, nuclei display moderate hyperchromasia, irregular chromatin distribution, and parachromatin clearing
Small to prominent nucleoli are present; nucleoli become larger with increasing grade of tumor
Cytoplasm is typically scant, cyanophilic, and often vacuolated
A watery, finely granular tumor diathesis is variably present.

Explanatory Notes and Diagnostic Problems
The above features are characteristic of the most common endometrioid type of adenocarcinoma. Cytologic detection of endometrial adenocarcinoma, especially well-differentiated tumors, in routinely prepared cervical/vaginal smears is limited by the low number of well-preserved abnormal cells and the subtlety of their cellular alterations. As compared with endocervical adenocarcinomas, endometrial carcinomas generally shed fewer cells, the cell size and nuclei are smaller, nucleoli are less prominent, and the tumor diathesis is watery rather than necrotic.

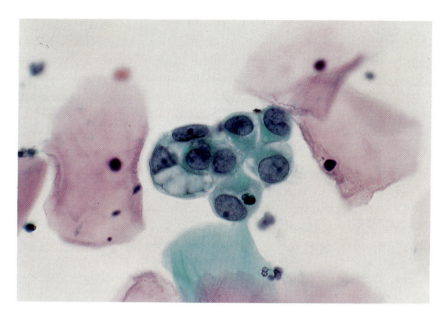

FIGURE 58. Endometrial adenocarcinoma.

Extrauterine Adenocarcinoma (Figs. 59,60):

When cells diagnostic of adenocarcinoma occur in association with a clean background or with morphology unusual for tumors of the uterus/cervix, an extrauterine neoplasm should be considered.

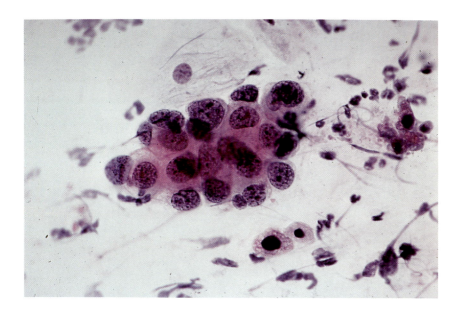

FIGURE 59. Metastatic breast carcinoma.

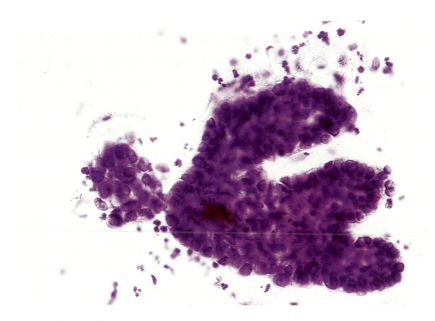

FIGURE 60. Papillary serous ovarian carcinoma.

Other Malignant Neoplasms

A wide variety of malignant tumors may be identified in cellular samples obtained from the cervix. One example is small cell undifferentiated (neuroendocrine) carcinoma (Fig. 61). The cytopathologist should provide as specific a diagnosis as possible to help guide the clinician in further evaluation of the patient.

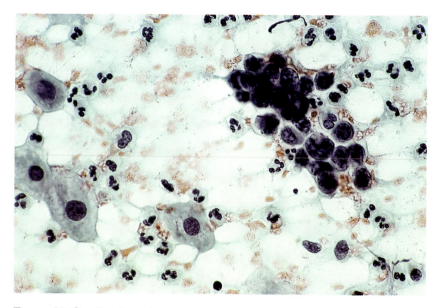

FIGURE 61. Small cell carcinoma.